Table of Contents

INTRODUCTION

You know that the food you eat does a lot more than just fill your belly — it can also provide you with energy, boost your mood, and lower your risk for several chronic

diseases. One of those diseases is cancer, the number 2
leading cause of death among Americans, per the
Centers for Disease Control and Prevention (CDC).
Smoothies can be a great way to add nutrition and
antioxidants to your diet to help with cancer prevention.
If you've already received a cancer diagnosis or have a
loved one who is fighting cancer, you might be
interested in this round-up of the best tips and recipes for
Cancer-Fighting Smoothies.

CHAPTER ONE

Overview

Learning that you have cancer can be stressful and
frightening. Knowing what to expect — from diagnosis
to recovery — can empower you and help you take
control of your health. This is a general overview of
what cancer is, symptoms to watch for, how it's
detected, treatments and post-treatment care.

What is cancer?

Cancer is a broad term. It describes the disease that
results when cellular changes cause the uncontrolled

growth and division of cells. Some types of cancer cause rapid cell growth, while others cause cells to grow and divide at a slower rate. Certain forms of cancer result in visible growths called tumors, while others, such as leukemia, do not. Most of the body's cells have specific functions and fixed lifespans. Cell death is part of a natural and beneficial phenomenon, which healthcare professionals call apoptosis. A cell receives instructions to die so that the body can replace it with a newer cell that functions better. Cancerous cells lack the components that instruct them to stop dividing and to die. As a result, they build up in the body, using oxygen and nutrients that would usually nourish other cells. Cancerous cells can form tumors, impair the immune system and cause other changes that prevent the body from functioning regularly. Cancerous cells may appear in one area, then spread via the lymph nodes. These are clusters of immune cells located throughout the body.

What is the difference between a normal cell and a cancerous cell?

Normally, cells follow instructions provided by genes. Genes set down rules for cells to follow, such as when to start and stop growing. Cancerous cells ignore the rules that normal cells follow:

• Normal cells divide and multiply in a controlled manner. Cancerous cells multiply uncontrollably.

• Normal cells are programmed to die (apoptosis). Cancerous cells ignore those directions.

• Normal cells for solid organs stay put. All cancerous cells are able to move around.

• Normal cells don't grow as fast as cancerous cells.

How does cancer start in my body?

Cancer starts when a gene or several genes mutate and create cancerous cells. These cells create cancer clusters, or tumors. Cancerous cells may break away from tumors, using your lymphatic system or bloodstream to travel to other areas of your body. For example, a tumor in your breast may spread to your lungs, making it hard for you to breathe. In some types of blood cancer, abnormal cells in your bone marrow make abnormal blood cells that multiply uncontrollably. Eventually, the abnormal cells crowd out normal blood cells.

According to the American Cancer Society, 1 in 2 men and people assigned male at birth (AMAB) and 1 in 3 women and people assigned female at birth (AFAB) will develop cancer. As of 2019, more than 16.9 million people in the U.S. were living with cancer. The most common cancers in the United States are:

• Breast cancer: Breast cancer is the most common type of cancer. It mostly affects women and people AFAB. But about 1% of all breast cancer cases affect men and people AMAB.

• Lung cancer: Lung cancer is the second most common cancer. There are two types of lung cancer: non-small cell cancer and small cell lung cancer.

• Prostate cancer: This cancer affects 1 in 9 men and people AMAB.

• Colorectal cancer: Colon cancer and rectal cancer affect different parts of your digestive system.

• Blood cancers: Leukemia and lymphoma are the most common blood cancers.

Almost anyone may develop cancer, but data show cancer cases vary based on race and sex. According to the 2022 Annual Report on Cancer, the disease:

• Affects slightly more men and people AMAB than women and people AFAB.

• Affects more Black men (AMAB) than people in other racial groups.

• Affects more women (AFAB) who are American Indian or Alaska natives than people in other racial groups.

• Almost anyone may develop cancer, but it typically affects people aged 60 and older.

Symptoms and Causes

What are cancer symptoms?

Cancer is a complicated disease. You can have cancer for years without developing symptoms. Other times, cancer may cause noticeable symptoms that get worse very quickly. Many cancer symptoms resemble other, less serious illnesses. Having certain symptoms doesn't mean you have cancer. In general, you should talk to a healthcare provider anytime there's a change in your body that lasts for more than two weeks.

First symptoms of cancer
Some common early cancer symptoms include:

• Unexplained weight loss.

• Chronic tiredness.

• Persistent pain.

• Fever that occurs mostly at night.

• Skin changes, particularly moles that change shape and size or new moles.

Left untreated, cancer may cause additional symptoms, including:

• Bruising or bleeding more easily.

• Lumps or bumps under your skin that don't go away.

• Difficulty breathing.

• Difficulty swallowing.

There are many causes of cancer, and some are preventable.

Preventable risk factors for cancer include:

• smoking

• heavy alcohol consumption

• excess body weight

• physical inactivity

• poor nutrition

• human papillomavirus infection

Other risk factors for cancer are not preventable. Currently, the most significant unpreventable risk factor is age. According to the American Cancer Society (ACS), doctors in the United States diagnose 88% of cancer cases in people ages 50 years or older.

Genetic factors can contribute to the development of cancer. A person's genetic code tells their cells when to divide and expire. Changes in the genes can lead to faulty instructions, and cancer can result. Genes also influence the cells' production of proteins, and proteins carry many of the instructions for cellular growth and division. Some genes change proteins that would usually repair damaged cells. This can lead to a predisposition for cancer. If a parent has these genes, they may pass on the altered instructions to their offspring. A doctor may refer to this as an inherited gene mutation. These mutations may contribute to the development of up to 10% of cancer cases. Some genetic mutations that increase the risk of developing cancer occur after birth. Healthcare professionals refer to these changes as "acquired gene mutations". Possible causes include smoking and sun exposure. These genetic changes cause cancer more commonly than inherited gene mutations. Other changes that can result in cancer take place in the chemical signals that determine how the cells turn specific genes on and off. Doctors may call these "epigenetic changes".

You can reduce your risk by changing some of your lifestyle choices:

• If you smoke or use tobacco, try to stop. Ask a healthcare provider about smoking cessation programs that can help you quit tobacco.

• Follow a diet plan that's healthy for you. If you want help managing your weight, ask a healthcare provider about nutritional guidance and weight management programs.

• Add exercise to your daily routine. Exercise may boost your immune system so it provides more protection against cancer.

• Avoid toxins, including asbestos, radon and pesticides.

• Protect yourself against sun damage.

• Have regular cancer screenings.

How do I recognize cancer before it starts to cause serious health problems?

Some cancers cause early symptoms, but others do not exhibit symptoms until they are more advanced. Many of these symptoms are often from causes unrelated to cancer. The best way to identify cancer early is to report any unusual, persistent symptoms to a doctor so they can offer advice about any further testing that may be needed.

Can people with cancer live a long life?

Each individual's outlook varies depending on the type of cancer they have and other factors, such as their overall health and whether the disease has spread. However, the ACS indicates that the overall cancer death rate has declined by 33% between 1991 and 2020.

How long can someone live with cancer without knowing?

Some types of cancer do not cause symptoms in the early stages. Therefore, a person may not know they are living with the disease until it reaches more advanced stages. For example, research indicates that carcinoid tumors may not present with any symptoms for years.

How do healthcare providers diagnose cancer?

Healthcare providers begin a cancer diagnosis by doing a comprehensive physical examination. They'll ask you to describe your symptoms. They may ask about your family medical history. They may also do the following tests:

• Blood tests.

• Imaging tests.

• Biopsies.

Blood tests

Blood tests for cancer may include:

• Complete blood count (CBC): A CBC test measures and counts your blood cells.

• Tumor markers: Tumor markers are substances that cancer cells release or that your normal cells release in response to cancer cells.

• Blood protein tests: Healthcare providers use a process called electrophoresis to measure immunoglobulins.

Your immune system reacts to certain cancers by releasing immunoglobulins.

• Circulating tumor cell tests: Cancerous tumors may shed cells. Tracking tumor cells helps healthcare providers monitor cancer activity.

Imaging tests

Imaging tests may include:

• Computed tomography (CT) scan: CT scans check for cancerous tumors' location and impact on your organs and bones.

• X-rays: X-rays use safe amounts of radiation to create images of your bones and soft tissues.

• Positron emission test (PET) scan: PET scans produce images of your organs and tissues at work. Healthcare providers may use this test to detect early signs of cancer.

• Ultrasound: An ultrasound uses high-intensity sound waves that show structures inside of your body.

• Magnetic resonance imaging (MRI): MRIs use a large magnet, radio waves and a computer to create images of your organs and other structures inside of your body.

• Iodine meta-iodobenzylguanidine (MIGB): This nuclear imaging test helps detect cancer, including carcinoid tumors and neuroblastoma.

Biopsies

A biopsy is a procedure healthcare providers do to obtain cells, tissue, fluid or growths that they'll examine under a microscope. There are several kinds of biopsies:

• Needle biopsy: This test may be called a fine needle aspiration or fine needle biopsy. Healthcare providers use a thin hollow needle and syringe to extract cells, fluid or tissue from suspicious lumps. Needle biopsies are often done to help diagnose breast cancer, thyroid cancer or cancer in your lymph nodes.

• Skin biopsy: Healthcare providers remove a small sample of your skin to diagnose skin cancer.

• Bone marrow biopsy: Healthcare providers remove a small sample of bone marrow so they can test the sample

for signs of disease, including cancer in your bone
marrow.

• Endoscopic or laparoscopic biopsy: These biopsies use
an endoscope or laparoscope to see the inside of your
body. With both of these methods, a small cut is made in
your skin and an instrument is inserted. An endoscope is
a thin, flexible tube with a camera on the tip, along with
a cutting tool to remove your sample. A laparoscope is a
slightly different scope.

• Excisional or incisional biopsy: For these open
biopsies, a surgeon cuts into your body and either the
entire tumor is removed (excisional biopsy) or a part of
the tumor is removed (incisional biopsy) to test or treat
it.

• Perioperative biopsy: This test may be called a frozen
section biopsy. This biopsy is done while you're having
another procedure. Your tissue will be removed and
tested right away. Results will come in soon after the
procedure, so if you need treatment, it can start
immediately.

Genetic testing

Cancer may happen when a single gene mutates or several genes that work together mutate. Researchers have identified more than 400 genes associated with cancer development. People who inherit these genes from their biological parents may have an increased risk of developing cancer. Healthcare providers may recommend genetic testing for cancer if you have an inherited form of cancer. They may also do genetic testing to do therapy that targets specific cancer genes. They use test results to develop a diagnosis. They'll assign a number or stage to your diagnosis. The higher the number, the more cancer has spread.

How is cancer stage determined?

Healthcare providers use cancer staging systems to plan treatment and develop a prognosis or expected outcome. TNM is the most widely used cancer staging system. T stands for primary tumor. N stands for lymph nodes and indicates whether a tumor has spread to your lymph nodes. M stands for metastasis, when cancer spreads.

Most cancers have four stages. The specific stage is determined by a few different factors, including the tumor's size and location:

• Stage I: The cancer is localized to a small area and hasn't spread to lymph nodes or other tissues.

• Stage II: The cancer has grown, but it hasn't spread.

• Stage III: The cancer has grown larger and has possibly spread to lymph nodes or other tissues.

• Stage IV: The cancer has spread to other organs or areas of your body. This stage is also referred to as metastatic or advanced cancer.

Though stages one through four are the most common, there's also a Stage 0. This earliest phase describes cancer that's still localized to the area in which it started. Cancers that are still in Stage 0 are usually easily treatable and are considered pre-cancerous by most healthcare providers.

Management and Treatment

How do healthcare providers treat cancer?

Doctors usually prescribe treatments based on the type of cancer, its stage at diagnosis, and the person's overall health.

Some examples of cancer treatment include:

• Chemotherapy aims to kill cancerous cells with medications that target rapidly dividing cells. The drugs can also help shrink tumors, but the side effects can be severe.

• Hormone therapy involves taking medications that change how certain hormones work or interfere with the body's ability to produce them. When hormones play a significant role, as with prostate and breast cancers, this is a common approach.

• Immunotherapy uses medications and other treatments to boost the immune system and encourage it to fight cancerous cells.

• Radiation therapy uses high-dose radiation to kill cancerous cells. Also, a doctor may recommend using radiation to shrink a tumor before surgery or reduce tumor-related symptoms.

• Stem cell transplant can be especially beneficial for people with blood-related cancers, such as leukemia or lymphoma. It involves removing cells, such as red or white blood cells, that chemotherapy or radiation has destroyed. Lab technicians then strengthen the cells and put them back into the body.

• Surgery is often a part of a treatment plan when a person has a cancerous tumor. Also, a surgeon may remove lymph nodes to reduce or prevent the disease's spread.

• Targeted therapies perform functions within cancerous cells to prevent them from multiplying. They can also boost the immune system. Two examples of these therapies are small-molecule drugs and monoclonal antibodies.

Doctors will often employ more than one type of treatment to maximize effectiveness.

If you're feeling nauseous or have an upset stomach from treatment, try adding in:

Plain yogurt. A good source of probiotics, which are gut-healthy bacteria.

Fresh mint. Try 4 to 6 leaves.

Freshly grated ginger. 2 teaspoons should do it.

Lemon zest. Half a teaspoon can act as a natural tummy soother.

Healthcare providers work to balance the treatment so it destroys cancer without harmful or lasting side effects. Even so, all cancer treatments have side effects. Some treatments cause side effects that last for years after treatment is completed. Many people benefit from palliative care that eases cancer symptoms and treatment side effects. The most common cancer treatment side effects are:

• Anemia.

• Nausea and vomiting.

• Fatigue.

• Pain.

What is the prognosis/outlook for cancer?

Improvements in cancer detection, increased awareness of the risks of smoking, and a drop in tobacco use have all contributed to a year-on-year decrease in the number of cancer diagnoses and deaths. According to the ACS, the overall cancer death rate declined by 33%Trusted Source between 1991 and 2020. When a person has cancer, their outlook will depend on whether the disease has spread and on its type, severity, and location.

Talk to your healthcare provider about any issues you experience while you're undergoing cancer treatment. Call your oncology team if you notice:

• A fever of 101 degrees Fahrenheit (38.33 degrees Celsius) or higher.

• Severe headaches.

• Chills.

• Persistent cough.

• Shortness of breath (dyspnea).

• Sores on your lips or in your mouth.

• Sudden weight loss greater than five pounds.

• Excessive vomiting (three times an hour for three hours or more).

• Blood in your urine (pee) or feces (poop).

• Excessive bleeding or bruising.

What questions should I ask my healthcare provider?
Knowledge is power. If you've been diagnosed with cancer, you'll want to gather as much information as you can. Here are some questions to ask your healthcare provider:

• What type of cancer do I have?

• Has the cancer spread to other areas of my body?

• Is my cancer genetic?

• What are my chances of survival?

• Which treatments do you recommend?

• What are the risks and benefits of my treatment?

• How long will treatment take?

• Will I be able to work during cancer treatment?

• Will cancer treatment affect my fertility?

• Will I need to stay in the hospital for my treatment?

• Would a clinical trial be a good option for me?

Anti-Cancer Healthy Smoothies

How do I make a healthy smoothie when I have cancer?

The following combinations make about 2 servings each.

Choose your liquid

Use 2 cups of one of the liquids below:

• Filtered water. A good choice for monitoring calories or making a milder tasting smoothie.

• Coconut water. A natural rehydration beverage, packed with electrolytes like sodium and potassium.

• Almond milk. This milk alternative is low-calorie and caffeine-free like water, but with a smooth silky texture.

• Low-fat milk. A great source of electrolytes with protein added to the mix.

• Fruit juice. A good choice for boosting calories or making a more robust, flavorful smoothie.

Try a mildly sweet fruit

Add 1 cup of slightly sweet, fiber-rich fruit to promote digestive health and to balance multiple flavors:

• Banana. A good source of potassium for healthy blood pressure and electrolyte balance.

• Ripe pear. A good source of flavonols, which are heart-healthy antioxidant plant compounds.

• Mango. An excellent source of immune-boosting vitamins A and C.

Include 1 cup of dark-colored fruit to take advantage of their cancer-fighting phytochemicals. These options all have heart-healthy antioxidant plant compounds:

• Berries or cherries. Good sources of anthocyanin.

• Watermelon. Good source of lycopene.

• Red or purple grapes. Good source of resveratrol.

Mix in some greens

Add 1 cup of tightly packed leafy greens to provide your body with B vitamins and iron to help reproduce blood cells, as well as other nutrients:

• Spinach. A power veggie known for iron, but also high in potent antioxidant vitamin A.

• Kale. A richly colored green and superfood high in antioxidant vitamins A and C.

• Romaine lettuce. High in vitamin A and a very mild in taste, it might be an appealing option if you've never tried greens in a smoothie before.

Choose a protein

Try adding in some protein to stabilize your blood sugar:

• Whole nuts or nut butters. Try adding 1 tablespoon of almonds, walnuts or natural peanut butter.

• Greek yogurt. Use 4 ounces of unsweetened Greek yogurt for a smooth finish.

• Protein powder. Add in 1/2 cup low-sugar protein powder. (Whey, hemp, rice or pea are all good options.)

Throw in some healthy fats

Did you know healthy fats help absorb nutrients as well as keep you feeling fuller, longer?

• Chia or flax seeds. Spoon in 1 teaspoon of chia or flax seeds, which aid in lowering blood pressure and are loaded with antioxidants, protein, iron and calcium.

• Avocado. Slice up 1 ripe avocado, which is high in oleic acid, an anti-inflammatory, as well as high in fiber.

• Coconut oil. Scoop 1 tablespoon of coconut oil into your smoothie, which is known to raise good cholesterol (HDL) and aid in heart health.

If you're looking for more ways to get your calorie count up, you can always add any of these ingredients:

• Ice cream. Choose one scoop of an ice cream flavor that blends well with the other ingredients in your smoothie.

• Olive oil. Add 1 tablespoon for a smoother, healthier smoothie. A drizzle a day keeps the doctor away!

• Honey. A healthier alternative to most smoothie sweeteners, try adding 1 tablespoon.

• Coconut cream. Another healthy fat that adds calories to your smoothie with just 1 tablespoon.

• Powdered milk. A great source of vitamin E, which aids in skin, nail and hair health. Scoop in 1 tablespoon.

CHAPTER TWO

Anti-Cancer Smoothie Recipes

Mango-Peach Smoothie

You can use fresh or frozen fruit in this yummy mango and peach smoothie. It tastes better if the fruit is frozen.

Prep Time: 10 mins

Total Time: 10 mins

Servings: 2

Ingredients

• 1 peach, sliced

• 1 mango, peeled and diced

• ½ cup vanilla soy milk

• ½ cup orange juice, or as needed

Directions

1. Place peach, mango, soy milk, and orange juice into a blender. Cover, and puree until smooth. Pour into glasses to serve.

Nutrition Facts (per serving)

105 Calories

1g Fat

22g Carbs

3g Protein

Quick, easy smoothies made entirely with fruit!

Prep Time: 10 mins

Total Time: 10 mins

Servings: 2

Yield: 2 servings

Ingredients

• 1 cup pineapple juice

• 1 large banana, cut into chunks

• 1 cup frozen strawberries

• 1 cup frozen blueberries

Directions

1. Pour pineapple juice into a blender and add banana, strawberries, and blueberries. Cover and blend until smooth, about 1 minute. Pour into 2 glasses.

Nutrition Facts (per serving)

205 Calories

1g Fat

51g Carbs

2g Protein

Start your day off right with this quick and nutritious apple smoothie, ready in minutes. This breakfast smoothie has a nice combination of fruit and is slightly sweet, creamy, and satisfying.

Prep Time: 5 mins

Cook Time: 0 mins

Total Time: 5 mins

Servings: 2

Ingredients

- 3/4 cup vanilla almond milk

- 1 apple - peeled, cored, and cubed

- 1 cup halved frozen strawberries

- 1 frozen banana, peeled and cubed

- 1/4 cup vanilla Greek yogurt (such as Cabot® 2% lowfat vanilla Greek yogurt)

Directions

1. Place almond milk, apple, strawberries, banana, and yogurt in a blender, being sure the milk goes in first. Process until smooth, occasionally scraping down the sides of the blender with a rubber spatula, if necessary.

2. Pour into serving glasses and serve immediately.

Nutrition Facts (per serving)

561 Calories

3g Fat

137g Carbs

9g Protein

Prep Time: 5 mins

Cook Time: 0 mins

Total Time: 5 mins

Servings: 1

Yield: 1 large smoothie

Ingredients

- 1 1/2 cups frozen blueberries

- 3/4 cup plain whole milk greek yogurt

- 1 handful fresh spinach, rinsed

- 1 banana

- 1/4 cup whole raw almonds

- 1 tablespoon ground flax

- 1 pinch ground cinnamon (optional)

- 1 pinch ground nutmeg (optional)

- 1 pinch ground cloves (optional)

- 1 pinch cardamom (optional)

- 2 tablespoons milk, or as needed

Directions

1. Place blueberries, Greek yogurt, spinach, banana, almonds, flax meal, cinnamon, nutmeg, cloves, and cardamom into a high-speed blender. Blend on high until smooth, 1 to 2 minutes. Add milk as needed to help it blend, and to achieve desired consistency.

Cook's Notes:

This smoothie is super adaptable to whatever ingredients you have on hand. You can use any frozen fruit you like; you can use almond butter in place of whole almonds; use any kind of yogurt or milk you prefer; and you can sweeten it with honey or maple syrup as needed.

This makes 1 very large serving and is meant to serve as a meal; however, it can easily be 2 servings if you prefer it as a snack. You may need to adjust how you blend this smoothie if you don't have a high-speed blender.

Nutrition Facts (per serving)

604 Calories

28g Fat

72g Carbs

26g Protein

A gorgeous indulgent pineapple smoothie with banana — simple, easy, and delicious!

Prep Time: 5 mins

Total Time: 5 mins

Servings: 1

Yield: 1 smoothie

Ingredients

• 4 ice cubes

• ¼ fresh pineapple - peeled, cored and cubed

• 1 large banana, cut into chunks

- 1 cup pineapple or apple juice

Directions

1. Gather all ingredients.

2. Place ice cubes, pineapple, banana, and pineapple juice into the container of a blender.

3. Purée on high until smooth.

4. Enjoy!

Nutrition Facts (per serving)

313 Calories

1g Fat

79g Carbs

3g Protein

Smoothies with a Boost

Look for kefir—a drinkable yogurt—in the refrigerated section near the milk and yogurt or in the specialty health sections of larger grocery stores.

Prep Time: 10 mins

Total Time: 10 mins

Servings: 2

Yield: 2 cups

Ingredients

- ½ cup kefir

- ½ cup cold brewed tea

- 1 cup frozen banana slices

- 1 cup frozen sliced strawberries

- 1 teaspoon matcha powder

Directions

1. Blend all ingredients in a blender until smooth, stopping to scrape down sides as needed, 2 to 3 minutes. Serve.

Cook's Notes:

You can use 1 cup of any frozen chopped or sliced fruit, any flavored kefir, and 1 to 2 teaspoon of any powder addition you like. You can use chilled brewed coffee instead of tea.

If you don't have frozen slices ready, swap in 1 ripe banana, sliced, and add 2 to 3 ice cubes.

Variations:

Pretty in Pink: Pomegranate-flavored kefir, white tea, sliced strawberries, and hibiscus powder (ground dried hibiscus flowers, found online)

Oh, Chai There: Vanilla-flavored kefir, black tea, chopped peaches, and chai tea powder

Matcha in Paradise: Coconut-flavored kefir, green tea, chopped mango, and matcha powder

Mocha-Cherry: Cherry-flavored kefir, coffee, pitted sweet cherries, and unsweetened cocoa powder

Nutrition Facts (per serving)

178 Calories

3g Fat

39g Carbs

4g Protein

This vegan oatmeal smoothie has a deep pink color and a rich, creamy texture. It's very filling, and perfect for people in a rush in the morning. You don't have to give up a good breakfast when it's this fast to make! I use vitamin fortified soy milk.

Prep Time: 5 mins

Total Time: 5 mins

Servings: 2

Ingredients

- 1 cup soy milk

- ½ cup rolled oats

- 14 frozen strawberries

- 1 banana, broken into chunks

- 1 ½ teaspoons white sugar (Optional)

- ½ teaspoon vanilla extract (Optional)

Directions

1. Gather ingredients.

2. Blend soy milk, oats, strawberries, and banana in a blender until smooth. Add sugar and vanilla and blend again until smooth.

3. Pour into glasses and serve.

Nutrition Facts (per serving)

142 Calories

4g Fat

21g Carbs

7g Protein

Creamy Banana Strawberry Split Smoothie

Prep Time: 10 mins

Total Time: 10 mins

Servings: 4

Yield: 4 servings

Ingredients

- 1 cup almond milk

- 1 chopped banana, frozen

- ¾ cup strawberries

- 3 ice cubes

- 1 scoop vanilla protein powder

- 1 teaspoon vanilla extract

- 1 teaspoon honey

- 1 teaspoon ground flax seed

- 1 teaspoon ground chia seeds

- ½ teaspoon ground cinnamon

Directions

1. Blend almond milk, banana, strawberries, ice cubes, protein powder, vanilla extract, honey, ground flax seeds, ground chia seeds, and cinnamon in a blender until smooth.

Nutrition Facts (per serving)

111 Calories

2g Fat

14g Carbs

10g Protein

This peanut butter banana smoothie is so refreshing, and it's sweet and tasty.

Prep Time: 5 mins

Total Time: 5 mins

Servings: 4

Yield: 4 servings

Ingredients

• 2 bananas, broken into chunks

• 2 cups milk

• ½ cup peanut butter

• 2 tablespoons honey, or to taste

• 2 cups ice cubes

Directions

1. Gather all ingredients.

2. Place bananas, milk, peanut butter, honey, and ice cubes in a blender.

3. Blend until smooth, about 30 seconds.

4. Enjoy!

Nutrition Facts (per serving)

335 Calories

19g Fat

34g Carbs

13g Protein

Banana, Avocado, and Spinach Smoothie

A quick and delicious banana, avocado, and spinach smoothie that can be used as a breakfast or snack!

Prep Time: 10 mins

Total Time: 10 mins

Servings: 2

Ingredients

• 1 banana, sliced

• ½ avocado, peeled and sliced

• ½ cup fresh spinach

• ½ cup 1% milk

• 6 ice cubes

• 2 teaspoons honey

• 1 teaspoon vanilla extract

Directions

1. Blend banana, avocado, spinach, milk, ice cubes, honey, and vanilla together in a blender until smooth.

Nutrition Facts (per serving)

190 Calories

8g Fat

28g Carbs

4g Protein

Prep Time: 5 mins

Total Time: 5 mins

Servings: 2

Yield: 2 servings

Ingredients

- ½ cup coconut milk

- ½ cup water, or more as needed

- ice cubes

- ½ medium avocado, pitted and scooped from shell

- ½ cup fresh spinach

- 2 tablespoons erythritol

- 1 tablespoon medium-chain triglyceride (MCT) oil

- ½ teaspoon vanilla powder

Directions

1. Combine coconut milk, water, ice cubes, avocado, spinach, erythritol, MCT oil, and vanilla powder in a blender. Blend until smooth.

Cook's Notes:

Feel free to replace coconut milk with 1/4 cup heavy whipping cream plus 1/4 cup water. You can substitute extra-virgin coconut oil for the MCT oil. Substitute 1 teaspoon vanilla extract for the vanilla powder if desired, and 5 to 8 drops of stevia extract instead of erythritol. Optional add-ins: 1/4 cup chocolate, vanilla, or plain whey protein, egg white protein powder (such as Jay Robb (R)), collagen powder, or plant-based NuZest(R).

Nutrition Facts (per serving)

256 Calories

26g Fat

18g Carbs

2g protein

Fig Smoothie
Prep Time: 5 mins

Total Time: 5 mins

Servings: 2

Ingredients

• 2 frozen bananas, peeled and chopped

• 6 fresh figs, halved

• ¾ cup milk

• ¾ cup orange juice

Directions

1. Place the bananas, figs, milk, and orange juice into a blender. Cover, and puree until smooth. Pour into glasses to serve.

Nutrition Facts (per serving)

335 Calories

3g Fat

78g Carbs

6g Protein

An energizing cucumber and pineapple smoothie with coconut water, ginger, and lemon.

Prep Time: 10 mins

Total Time: 10 mins

Servings: 1

Ingredients

• 1 cup coconut water, or to taste

• 1 cup chopped fresh pineapple

• 1 stalk celery

• ½ cucumber, peeled

• ½ lemon, peeled

• ⅓ bunch fresh parsley

• 1 (1 inch) piece fresh ginger root

Directions

1. Gather all ingredients.

2. Blend coconut water, pineapple, celery, cucumber, lemon, parsley, and ginger together in a blender until smooth.

Nutrition Facts (per serving)

169 Calories

1g Fat

43g Carbs

5g Protein

Frozen Berry Smoothie

Prep Time: 5 mins

Total Time: 5 mins

Servings: 1

Yield: 1 smoothie

Ingredients

• 1 cup milk

• 1 cup frozen berries (marionberries, raspberries, and blueberries)

• 2 tablespoons dark brown sugar

• 2 tablespoons white grape juice

• 1 teaspoon vanilla extract

• 1 ice cube

Directions

1. Combine milk, berries, brown sugar, grape juice, vanilla extract, and ice cube in a blender; blend until smooth.

Nutrition Facts (per serving)

317 Calories

5g Fat

60g Carbs

9g Protein

Almond Berry Smoothie

Almond milk and almond butter are the star ingredients in this berry smoothie with almond milk for a nutritious, on-the-go meal that is vegan and paleo-friendly.

Prep Time: 10 mins

Total Time: 10 mins

Servings: 1

Ingredients

- 1 cup frozen blueberries

- 1 banana

- ½ cup almond milk

- 1 tablespoon almond butter

- water as needed

Directions

1. Combine blueberries, banana, almond milk, and almond butter in a blender; blend until smooth, adding water for a thinner smoothie.

Cook's Note:

Any type of frozen berry can be used in place of the blueberries, if desired.

Nutrition Facts (per serving)

321 Calories

12g Fat

56g Carbs

5g Protein

Prep Time: 10 mins

Total Time: 10 mins

Servings: 4

Yield: 4 servings

Ingredients

• 1 banana, broken into chunks

• 3 whole frozen strawberries, or more to taste

• ¾ cup milk

• ½ cup plain yogurt

• ¼ cup pumpkin puree

• 2 tablespoons creamy peanut butter

- 1 tablespoon brown sugar

- ¼ teaspoon ground cinnamon (Optional)

- 1 pinch ground nutmeg

- 8 ice cubes, or as desired

- ¼ cup whipped cream, or more to taste (Optional)

- 1 pinch ground cinnamon (Optional)

Directions

1. Blend banana, strawberries, milk, yogurt, pumpkin puree, peanut butter, brown sugar, 1/4 teaspoon cinnamon, and nutmeg in a blender until smooth; add ice cubes and again blend until smooth. Pour smoothie into 4 glasses and top with whipped cream and a pinch of cinnamon.

Nutrition Facts (per serving)

149 Calories

7g Fat

19g Carbs

6g Protein

This healthy fruit smoothie with raspberries, blueberries, strawberries, and more is absolutely wonderful!

Prep Time: 5 mins

Total Time: 5 mins

Servings: 2

Ingredients

- ⅓ cup fresh blueberries

- ⅓ cup fresh raspberries

- 4 large fresh strawberries, hulled

- ⅔ cup milk

- ⅓ cup pomegranate juice

- ⅓ cup mango juice

- 2 tablespoons honey

Directions

1. Place berries into a blender with milk, pomegranate and mango juices, and honey. Cover and purée until smooth. Pour into glasses to serve.

Nutrition Facts (per serving)

191 Calories

2g Fat

43g Carbs

3g Protein

Mint and Fruit Smoothie

This quick, frosty blender recipe has a thick texture, beautiful colors, and a fruity, mojito-like taste.

Prep Time: 10 mins

Total Time: 10 mins

Servings: 2

Yield: 2 cups

Ingredients

• ¼ cup red seedless grapes, frozen

- ¼ cup unsweetened applesauce, or to taste

- 1 tablespoon fresh lime juice

- 3 frozen strawberries

- 1 cup cubed fresh pineapple

- 3 fresh mint leaves

Directions

1. Place frozen grapes, applesauce, and lime juice into a blender. Puree until smooth. Add frozen strawberries, cubed pineapple, and mint leaves. Pulse a few times until the strawberries and pineapple are in small bits.

Nutrition Facts (per serving)

92 Calories

0g Fat

24g Carbs

1g Protein

This is a great smoothie for breakfast - and sometimes dinner! You can substitute the orange juice with any mix of juices or even soy milk! The soy milk adds more of a milk shake quality than the juice does.

Prep Time: 5 mins

Total Time: 5 mins

Servings: 5

Yield: 4 to 6 drinks

Ingredients

• 2 frozen bananas, skins removed and cut in chunks

• ½ cup frozen blueberries

• 1 cup orange juice

• 1 tablespoon honey (Optional)

• 1 teaspoon vanilla extract (Optional)

Directions

1. Place bananas, blueberries and juice in a blender, puree. Use honey and/or vanilla to taste. Use more or less liquid depending on the thickness you want for your smoothie.

Nutrition Facts (per serving)

88 Calories

0g Fat

21g Carbs

1g Protein

Mixed Fruit Smoothie with Goji Berries

Prep Time: 5 mins

Total Time: 5 mins

Servings: 1

Ingredients

• 1 cup frozen mixed fruit

• 1 cup vanilla soy milk

• 2 tablespoons dried goji berries

- 1 teaspoon honey

Directions

1. Place mixed fruit, soy milk, goji berries, and honey into a blender; process until smooth.

Tips

Preferably silk vanilla soy milk, but you can just as easily use almond milk or swap it for water and a frozen banana. You will want to blend longer than a regular smoothie to ensure the goji berries are liquified.

Nutrition Facts (per serving)

341 Calories

5g Fat

66g Carbs

12g Protein

Healthy Fruit and Vegetable Smoothie

A great mix of fruits and vegetables to get started in the morning or post workout that still tastes awesome.

Prep Time: 10 mins

Total Time: 10 mins

Servings: 1

Yield: 1 smoothie

Ingredients

• 6 fluid ounces milk

• 1 (6 ounce) container plain yogurt

• ½ cup frozen strawberries

• ½ frozen banana

• ¼ cup frozen blueberries

• 1 green ice cube (see footnote)

• 2 tablespoons whey protein powder (Optional)

• 1 teaspoon honey, or to taste

Directions

1. Combine milk, yogurt, strawberries, banana, blueberries, green ice cube, whey, and honey in a blender, in the order listed. Blend until smooth.

Cook's Notes:

To Make the Veggie ice cube, you'll need a bunch of kale(stems removed and discarded), a package of spinach, and 1 large avocado. Blanch the kale and spinach in a pot of boiling water until wilted, about 1 minute. Strain the leaves and put in a food processor with avocado; blend until smooth. Pour mixture into ice cube trays and freeze.

Nutrition Facts (per serving)

372 Calories

7g Fat

63g Carbs

18g Protein

Orange Banana Smoothie

Prep Time: 10 mins

Total Time: 10 mins

Servings: 2

Ingredients

- 1 cup cold milk

- ½ cup vanilla fat-free yogurt

- ¼ cup sugar

- 1 pinch salt

- 2 medium oranges, peeled and segmented

- 1 medium banana

- 4 cubes ice

Directions

1. Gather all ingredients.

2. Combine milk, yogurt, sugar, and salt in a blender. Add oranges and banana and blend for about 1 minute. Add ice and blend until smooth.

3. Serve and enjoy!

Nutrition Facts (per serving)

340 Calories

3g Fat

74g Carbs

9g Protein

Prep Time: 5 mins

Total Time: 5 mins

Servings: 2

Yield: 2 servings

Ingredients

- 1 ½ cups ice cubes

- 1 cup fresh raspberries

- 1 cup orange juice

- 1 banana, cut into chunks

- ½ cup vanilla fat-free yogurt

- 1 teaspoon honey, or to taste

Directions

65

1. Blend ice cubes, raspberries, orange juice, banana, yogurt, and honey in a blender until smooth.

Nutrition Facts (per serving)

206 Calories

1g Fat

47g Carbs

5g Protein

Kiwi Banana Apple Smoothie

This smoothie is tasty and super-healthy - a lot of thanks to the seeds and powder used in it.

Prep Time: 10 mins

Total Time: 10 mins

Servings: 2

Yield: 2 servings

Ingredients

• 1 apple, roughly chopped

• 1 banana, broken into chunks

- 2 kiwifruit, peeled

- 1 ¼ cups milk

- ¼ cup ice, or as desired

- 2 teaspoons chia seeds

- 1 teaspoon maca powder

Directions

1. Blend apple, banana, kiwifruit, milk, ice, chia seeds, and maca powder together in a blender until smooth.

Nutrition Facts (per serving)

232 Calories

5g Fat

44g Carbs

8g Protein

Breakfast Banana Green Smoothie

Easy and simple, you'll have this smoothie in no time. This smoothie is packed with nutrients and vitamins. It's also perfect if you're in a hurry to get to work, or just craving a fresh and healthy drink to start your day. Organic maple syrup can be added instead of honey.

Prep Time: 5 mins

Total Time: 5 mins

Servings: 1

Yield: 1 serving

Ingredients

• 2 cups baby spinach leaves, or to taste

• 1 banana

• 1 carrot, peeled and cut into large chunks

• ¾ cup plain fat-free Greek yogurt, or to taste

• ¾ cup ice

• 2 tablespoons honey

Directions

1. Put spinach, banana, carrot, yogurt, ice, and honey in a blender; blend until smooth.

Nutrition Facts (per serving)

367 Calories

1g Fat

77g Carbs

19g Protein

Veggies, fruit, and milk all in 1 drink! Plus it's 'skinny'!

Prep Time: 5 mins

Total Time: 5 mins

Servings: 2

Yield: 2 servings

Ingredients

• 2 cups fresh spinach

• 2 cups frozen strawberries

• 1 frozen banana

• 1 ½ cups unsweetened almond milk

• 1 tablespoon agave nectar (Optional)

Directions

1. Combine spinach, strawberries, banana, almond milk, and agave in a blender; blend until smooth.

Nutrition Facts (per serving)

190 Calories

3g Fat

43g Carbs

3g Protein

This is a refreshing smoothie that will help get your fruit and vegetable servings in for the day. You can use this recipe and just substitute the fruits you like and the greens you want for that day. You could use juice instead of water, if desired.

Prep Time: 15 mins

Total Time: 15 mins

Servings: 2

Yield: 36 ounces

Ingredients

• 2 cups frozen strawberries

• 1 ½ cups warm water

• 2 cups milk

• 1 ½ cups fresh spinach, or to taste

• 1 cup frozen blueberries

• 1 frozen chopped banana

• 1 tablespoon honey

• ½ lemon, juiced

Directions

1. Place strawberries in a bowl; add warm water.

2. Blend milk and spinach together in a blender until smooth. Add blueberries, banana, and honey and blend until smooth. Add strawberries-water mixture and lemon juice and blend until smooth.

Nutrition Facts (per serving)

303 Calories

6g Fat

57g Carbs

10g Protein

Watermelon Refreshing Green Smoothie
Prep Time: 10 mins

Total Time: 10 mins

Servings: 1

Ingredients

• 2 cups diced watermelon

• ½ cup fresh spinach

• ¼ cup broccoli florets

• ¼ cucumber, sliced

• ½ apple - peeled, cored, and diced, or more to taste

• 1 stalk celery, coarsely chopped

Directions

1. Place watermelon in a blender; mix until liquefied. Add spinach, broccoli, cucumber, apple, and celery; blend until smooth.

Nutrition Facts (per serving)

64 Calories

0g Fat

15g Carbs

2g Protein

Beet Smoothie

This delicious beet smoothie is a gorgeous color and naturally sweet thanks to beets, pineapple, and banana.

Prep Time: 15 mins

Total Time: 15 mins

Servings: 2

Yield: 2 smoothies

Ingredients

• 2 medium beets, scrubbed

- 1 green apple

- 1 avocado, peeled and pitted

- ¾ cup fresh pineapple chunks

- 1 banana, peeled

- ice cubes

Directions

1. Juice beets and green apples, including peels, in an electric juicer.

2. Combine apple-beet juice, avocado, pineapple, banana, and ice in a high-speed blender; blend until smooth.

Nutrition Facts (per serving)

310 Calories

15g Fat

47g Carbs

5g Protein

This chocolate and strawberry smoothie made with bananas and yogurt is a wonderful treat for any occasion.

Prep Time: 5 mins

Total Time: 5 mins

Servings: 2

Ingredients

• 2 bananas, cut into chunks and frozen

• ½ cup frozen strawberries

• 2 tablespoons chocolate syrup

• 1 cup plain yogurt

Directions

1. In a blender, combine bananas, strawberries, chocolate syrup, and yogurt. Blend until smooth.

Nutrition Facts (per serving)

248 Calories

3g Fat

51g Carbs

8g Protein

This quick green smoothie provides what you need for a fruity, veggie snack—with spinach, banana, pineapple, and almondmilk.

Prep Time: 5 mins

Total Time: 5 mins

Servings: 1

Yield: 1 smoothie

Ingredients

• 1 cup baby spinach leaves

• 1 banana, cut into chunks

• ½ cup pineapple chunks

• ¾ cup Almond Breeze Original or Unsweetened Original almondmilk

Directions

1. Place all ingredients into blender and blend on high until smooth.

Nutrition Facts (per serving)

130 Calories

2g Fat

28g Carbs

2g Protein

A tasty green smoothie that is sure to please. Get your fruit and veggie servings before heading out the door.

Prep Time: 5 mins

Total Time: 5 mins

Servings: 1

Yield: 1 smoothie

Ingredients

• ½ cup spinach

• ½ pear, chopped

• ½ lemon, juiced

• 1 cup Almond Breeze Original almondmilk

Directions

1. Place all ingredients into blender and blend on high until smooth.

Cook's Notes:

Easily swap Almond Breeze Almondmilk 1:1 for any recipe that calls for dairy milk. Feel free to substitute in your favorite Almond Breeze almondmilk flavor (Vanilla, Chocolate, Unsweetened Original, Unsweetened Vanilla, Unsweetened Chocolate, Blended with Real Bananas, Coconut Almond blend, or Cashew Almond Blend).

Nutrition Facts (per serving)

122 Calories

2g Fat

27g Carbs

4g Protein

78

A creamy, peach and orange smoothie is layered on top of a strawberry smoothie--pretty as a picture and oh so delicious.

Prep Time: 10 mins

Total Time: 10 mins

Servings: 2

Yield: 2 servings

Ingredients

- 1 cup frozen strawberries

- 1 large banana, peeled and halved

- 1 (5.3 ounce) container Yoplait® Greek 100 Vanilla Yogurt, divided

- ¼ cup milk

- 1 tablespoon honey

- 1 cup sliced frozen peaches

- ¼ cup orange juice

Directions

1. Combine the strawberries, half the banana, 1/2 container of yogurt, milk and honey (if using) in a blender and blend until smooth. Pour into 2 glasses and rinse out the blender.

2. Combine the remaining half the banana, remaining yogurt, peaches and orange juice in the blender and blend until smooth. Pour over the strawberry smoothie layer and serve.

Nutrition Facts (per serving)

235 Calories

1g Fat

46g Carbs

10g Protein

Fresh Peach Trifle

This trifle with peaches is one of the best desserts. Although it takes a little work, the results can be described with one word: yummy!

Prep Time: 30 mins

Total Time: 30 mins

Servings: 8

Ingredients

• 6 large ripe peaches - peeled, pitted, and sliced

• 1 tablespoon fresh lemon juice

• 2 (8 ounce) containers vanilla yogurt

• 1 teaspoon lemon zest

• 1 (10 inch) prepared angel food cake, cut into cubes

Directions

1. Place peach slices into a large bowl and gently toss with lemon juice. Transfer 1 cup peaches to a blender and blend until smooth; set remaining peach slices aside.

2. Stir puréed peaches, yogurt, and lemon zest together in a bowl until well blended.

3. Layer 1/2 of the cake cubes in the bottom of a glass dish. Top with 1/2 of the peach slices, then 1/2 of the

yogurt mixture, then all of the remaining cake cubes. Arrange the remaining peaches over top, reserving five or six slices for garnish. Cover with the remaining yogurt mixture, then arrange the reserved peach slices over top. Refrigerate until ready to serve.

Nutrition Facts (per serving)

182 Calories

1g Fat

38g Carbs

5g Protein

Lemon-Raspberry Trifle

This lemon-raspberry trifle is a great summer dessert to share at gatherings.

Prep Time: 20 mins

Cook Time: 5 mins

Additional Time: 20 mins

Total Time: 45 mins

Servings: 18

Yield: 1 large trifle

Ingredients

Simple Syrup:

• ¾ cup water

• 1 cup white sugar

• ¼ cup lemon juice

• 1 large lemon, zested

Trifle:

• 3 (6 ounce) containers fresh raspberries

• 1 (8 ounce) container frozen whipped topping (such as Cool Whip®), thawed

• 4 tablespoons lemon curd

• 4 cups prepared vanilla pudding

• 1 (16 ounce) prepared pound cake, cut into cubes

Directions

1. Stir sugar and water for simple syrup together in a saucepan over medium heat until sugar is dissolved. Let cool, about 20 minutes, then stir in lemon juice and lemon zest.

2. Toss raspberries in a bowl with 2 tablespoons simple syrup. Set aside about 3 ounces berries for top of trifle.

3. Gently fold together whipped topping and lemon curd. Add to the vanilla pudding and fold until incorporated.

4. In a large trifle bowl, layer 1/3 of the pound cake cubes. Spoon a couple teaspoons simple syrup over the cake layer, then add 1/3 of the berries and 1/3 of the pudding mixture. Repeat layers twice more, then scatter reserved berries on top.

Cook's Notes:

You really can't mess this recipe up. Change up the berries or amount of lemon to your taste. Warning: Do not add of all the simple syrup; it will make it too soggy.

Nutrition Facts (per serving)

290 Calories

10g Fat

48g Carbs

3g Protein

Smoothies are a good option if your treatment gives you side effects. Smoothies are also cold, which can soothe a sore mouth and throat. If you're just too tired to eat, or you don't have an appetite, drinking your calories may be an easy alternative. However, it's important to keep in mind that nutrition is very individualized for everyone, especially for those with cancer. Smoothie recipes should be modified based on your preferences.